my
hundred
helpers

my
hundred
helpers

THE PROVISION OF GOD
THROUGH PEOPLE

Jeff Hopper

LINKS PLAYERS PUBLISHING
A ministry of Links Players International
La Quinta, California

my hundred helpers

Links Players International is a mission organization presenting the gospel of Jesus Christ to all who will hear. Our specific calling is to change the conversation where people play golf. Find out more at linksplayers.com.

Cover photos:
Front: XiXinXing (istockphoto.com)
Back: Ales Otuvko (istockphoto.com)

Other books by Jeff Hopper:
Go for the Green
The Red Door Community (with Jeffrey Cranford)
Love Never Fails (with Jeffrey Cranford)

To my wife, Laura,
my helper at all times

and to the Lord Jesus Christ,
whose healing in this life
is only a whisper of what is to come

table of contents

for starters

I HAVE NO DESIRE TO BE THE CANCER GUY. I certainly didn't want this before I had cancer, and I don't want it now.

But I know three things to be true, and they have set me up for this little book you are about to read.

First, God will do what he will do. You don't have to be a Bible scholar to know this, but a tour through the Scriptures will plant this truth in you. God, in all his constancy, remains rather unpredictable. Or, you might say, just when you get to thinking you're quite comfortable where you are, you can expect God to kick you off the couch.

Second, one of the things God has done is make a writer of me. While I enjoyed my first two years of college, and particularly the opportunity they gave me to continue playing competitive golf, they also exposed me to the world of journalism. So I transferred colleges ahead of my junior year to a school that didn't have a golf team, but which immediately gave me a chance to do the sports reporting I wanted to do and to write a number of other things as well. I had mentors at both schools. It was a Chinese history professor on the first campus who began to teach me that verbosity only goes so far before it detracts from the main point. At my second stop, a young instructor who probably had no business bearing that title, gave us budding writers his heart and soul and produced a willingness to work late into the night and a hunger to "get it right." And because this was a school that required a heavy dose of biblical instruction to go along with our major, I was also writing theology papers and sharing time with missionaries and ministers. Our little pool of writers has produced a major voice in the Reformed movement (Michael Horton), a widely read Hollywood reporter (Glenn Whipp), and a guy who has spent seventeen years now writing nearly every day about the curious connection between God and golf (me).

Finally, I am well aware of the adage that says writers write best when they write from their experience. My longtime partner in ministry, Jeffrey Cranford, puts it like this: "You cannot give out what you do not possess." So now, despite my lack of desire for such a fate, I possess cancer. Perhaps. The doctors did a fantastic job at getting it out (more on that later!), and my wife and I have been praying that any residual cancer cells are put to death by God himself. At the time of this writing in mid-2017, it's too early to tell what's all there and what's gone for good, but the first two rotations of scans have come back clear. Maybe God has already answered our prayers in the way we have asked them. Either way, cancer and its treatments are woven into the words on the pages ahead. I have been told that my writing since cancer is "richer," "more insightful," things like that. Frankly, I can't tell the difference. My method hasn't changed: I sit down and start moving my fingers. And my message is pretty much the same: God is in charge, and it's a very good thing he is, because I would have messed things up beyond repair by now if I were going it on my own.

I think you will find that this book is written with two tones. I didn't set out to highlight my cancer so much, but in opening that door, it has been a help to others. I write those words quite personally, of course, and maybe more poetically (you can be the judge of that).

My original intention though was to convey the core of two sermons I preached in late 2016 through the form in front of you now. I want to show you how God supplies your needs and how he does so most often through the people he brings into your life. The most beautiful words a teacher or writer can hear are that someone who has heard your message or read your words has found application for the things you have written. This happened several times over after delivering those sermons. To me this suggested that what I had to say was meaningful to a full range of people, not just those who have experienced something as daunting as cancer.

Overall, you may find that portions of this book will sound instructive while other parts are narrative. To blend the two tones might do damage to both, so I've left them side-by-side, trusting you'll recognize the difference.

So here we go. Let me introduce you to my hundred helpers—and yours.

Jeff Hopper
Summer 2017

the year of my cancer

Just before Thanksgiving 2015, my wife told me a story she had heard from friends at the hospital where she works as a nurse. It was a celebrity story, not the kind she usually comes home and tells, but it had a weighty aspect to it.

For several years, Tarek and Christina El Moussa headlined a series on HGTV called *Flip or Flop*, a show my wife and I sometimes watched. One evening in 2013 a registered nurse was watching the program and, thanks to high definition, noticed that something was not right about Tarek's neck. There was a lump that didn't belong. The nurse, Ryan Reade, contacted the show's producers to suggest that Tarek see a doctor. Reade's suspicions were right; Tarek had thyroid cancer. He was treated and survived.

I suppose you tell your spouse these kinds of stories as a precaution, just as you might remind each other to get your mammograms, PSA tests, or colonoscopies (I know, this is not the romantic side of marriage). In this case, Laura's storytelling may have saved my life. She was the first of my hundred helpers.

A day or two later I stood in front of the mirror doing my morning shaving, and I noticed something shocking. My Adam's apple was far off center. How I had never seen it before, I do not know. I guess I had never had reason to look. Now it was unmistakable.

I didn't need Laura's urging to see the doctor, though this was something I rarely did as a typically healthy 52-year-old. I made an appointment. So unusual were my visits that I was pushed over to a new doctor in the clinic. He was caring and helpful and you'll hear more of him later, but what you need to know at this stage is that he agreed my condition was far out of the ordinary; he ordered scans.

On Christmas Eve, the doctor called. They had found a mass, maybe two, in my neck and chest. He scheduled me with specialists, who ordered biopsies and eventually set me up to meet with a surgeon at Stanford Medical Center. Stanford is three hours from my home, but it is common for the serious cases from our area to be sent there. The ENT specialist just three blocks from my house was passing me on, but she did so because she knew two things: the intricacy of the mass in my neck was beyond her comfort level and the surgeon she was sending me to, with whom she had worked at MD Anderson Medical Center in Houston, was world class. Now we were into 2016, and my appointment was scheduled for January 29. To ease the tension of the trip, I made reservations at a favorite restaurant near Palo Alto.

THE FIRST TIME I MET DR. CHRIS HOLSINGER, he put me off. I don't mean there was something about him that bugged me—not in the least. What I mean is that he stepped into the room where we waited for him, introduced himself, then said, "I'll be back in few minutes. I need to go next door and look at your scans." So we tapped our feet a bit longer.

When he returned, he threw open the door and summed up my condition with words I'll probably never forget:

"Wow, that's impressive!" We laughed, which was a good thing. Besides the structural compromise, though, the news appeared to be positive. Probably not cancer, but a large lipomous tumor (a fatty mass). Still, he wanted another biopsy, CT-guided this time and there at Stanford. As they say, just to be sure.

The schedulers set me up for the biopsy and then a return visit on February 29. When I had first heard word of the mass, indications were that a surgery would happen in January to get it out. We were quickly leaving that date behind. Not for the last time, we had to trust that the doctors had a better sense of the urgency than we did. And maybe since I was not being put on the fast track, we could take this as a hopeful sign.

The biopsy demanded a bit more of me than previous punches had. The Stanford team wanted to get it right. They used laser guidance to go deeper into the tumor and draw out more samples. Still, I had no suspicions of cancer. Something worse, maybe—a desmoid tumor, which is rare and by itself harmless but nearly inoperable because of its invasive threading. But the concerns here came only from my Google research, not from anything the doctors said. I didn't even want to mention this to Laura. We did little scouring of the internet, which can quickly drop you into an abyss of fear. Mostly we waited to hear whatever news would come from the mouths of the experts themselves.

We returned to Stanford on that extra day in February and even before the doctor stepped in, the nurse practitioner asked the question that in other cases might have "changed everything." He said, "Has anyone told you you have cancer?" He posed it this way, thinking someone may have already informed us over the phone. No one had. Here was the first time we had been given the news.

Forgive me if this kills the suspense, but I think it will help to say right up front that the cancer I have, as we confirmed through the course of the year with post-op biopsies and genetic tests, is as non-scary as it gets. It's also quite rare. I had—may still have—a well-differentiated liposarcoma. Such tumors develop in only one person per 200,000, but they usually grow in the thigh or less frequently in the abdomen. To have a liposarcoma in the neck and mediastinum (upper chest cavity) is beyond unusual. But for all the intricacies of the tumor's location, the cells of this cancer are non-metastizing and extremely slow-growing. The danger was in the tumor's size and the compromising of key structures being done by its growth. Fill a water bottle to the brim and stick it in the freezer and you're going to have problems; something's got to give. This is what was happening in my neck, where this tumor had wormed its way between my esophagus and trachea.

Other than the visual reference of my displaced Adam's apple, the only symptom I had of the tumor was shortness of breath over the previous year. But I had reason to ignore it, because every time I exercised I would actually breathe much better. A few months before the diagnosis I played 90 minutes of ultimate frisbee at 5,000 feet with a bunch of men quite younger than me; I had outlasted nearly all of them. What could be wrong? Now, as the results of my tests kept supplying more information, I knew: Strong exercise improved the passage of air through my crooked windpipe.

There is a name for the team that prepares and dispenses care for a cancer patient like me: the tumor board. It's a bit funny to think that these surgeons and oncologists and radiologists come together each week to talk tumors. Not your typical conversation among friends. Now I was on their docket. *What will we do with Mr. Hopper?*

The initial plan was to go to surgery, a couple weeks into March. That thinking held only for a few days. At the next gathering of the tumor board, Dr. Holsinger expressed that he wasn't sure the surgery would be successful enough without radiation. The problem was margin. When a tumor grows in one's thigh or abdomen, there is normally a layer of fat or muscle (or both) surrounding the mass. Surgeons cut out some of fat or muscle around the tumor, taking a margin of what they hope will be entirely non-cancerous material. If this margin is clean, no cancer cells are left in the body. But what if the tumor is pressed up against structures that have no fat or muscle, such as the esophagus or trachea? The idea is that with a regimen of radiation, a crust of dead cells can be created along the outside of the tumor. Doctors are in essence building the margin.

By now you may have guessed that the number of my helpers was increasing almost daily. A thoracic surgeon, Dr. Mark Berry, was already on board. His role would be to initiate the surgery from below—between my ribs—and free the tumor from its attachments in the mediastinum, including the area just above my heart. Then Dr. Holsinger would make the incision in my neck, gradually work the tumor out from the danger zones, and in the end lift the tumor up out of my chest. Now both these men were put on hold.

I should stop here to let you in on two more details: the size and nature of the tumor. The tumor itself, confirmed to be almost certainly just one growth, was the size and rough shape of two hands pressed together and held upright in the classic pose of prayer. The lower, thicker part was less dense, positioned as it was with more room to grow. Its character showed it to be a lipoma, a spontaneously developing fatty deposit that is quite common, though again unusual in the upper chest. Higher up that lipoma had taken a turn, however, transitioning to this cancer we call liposarcoma. There it was far denser, and it was this firmness that was giving it strength to start bullying the tender structures of the neck. How long had this tumor been growing? Dr. Holsinger speculated as long as twenty years!

Cancer, once it is identified, becomes the work of an oncologist. For me this was Dr. Kristen Ganjoo, who often was tasked with the role of explaining the worst of it when it came to what I was facing. She possessed a meaningful compassion to go along with this unhappy job, and there was never a day we didn't appreciate her optimism. Still, chemotherapy is a nasty business and she had to explain that my program of treatment, wherein the chemotherapy would be used to augment the radiation, would look like this: five days in hospital receiving ifosfamide while at the same time receiving a dose of radiation each of those days. Then a weekend off, followed by two more sets of weekdays coming in for radiation treatments. The fourth week I would return to the hospital for more chemotherapy, never skipping a beat in the radiation days, which ran for a fifth week before coming to a halt.

The radiation introduced another remarkable aspect of the treatment. Here the helper was Dr. Lynn Million, a radiation oncologist who was called on to prepare my body for the two minutes of application each day that would kill enough cells that the surgery could finally go forward. The treatments to be used made my insurance company balk: intensity-modulated radiation therapy. Throughout my care, there were helpers I never met. When it came to radiation, this was the team of engineers who worked with the doctor to design the dosage of the radiation and the pinpointing aim of the machine that would do the work. I did meet the techs who strapped me in for my rehearsal and created the mask that, with its eight or ten snaps, would hold my head to the table and make it immovable during the treatments.

What a wonder of technology all this was. The mask it-self was plastic mesh, warmed to make it soft, then pressed down over my face to mold it over my nose and mouth, down over my ears and head and neck, then flattened with flanges so it could be secured to the table. Each morning I was met by two or three women assigned to lay me down, lock me in, then step behind the barrier and start the machine. Our meetings were matters of serious business, but our greetings were always warm, often including some exchange about the Golden State Warriors, where much talk leaned in the Bay Area in those days as the team closed in on the record for most wins in the NBA's regular season then moved toward the playoffs. It would take fifteen or twenty minutes to set me up and run the radiation and any other scans that needed to happen that day, though the actual dose only lasted those two brief minutes. In the beginning, this was all exceedingly fasci-nating and probably came with an extra shot of adrenalin; by the final two or three days, it became nearly unbearable. I was having trouble swallowing and encountered intense crippling headaches right behind my left cheekbone. These were brief, but if they came at the wrong time, it was all I could do to sit up.

In the midst of writing this book, I saw an episode of *Fe-herty*, a show on the Golf Channel where former European Tour professional David Feherty interviews notables in and around the game. His guest for this particular show was Hall of Famer Phil Mickelson, whose wife and mother were diag-nosed with breast cancer within months of one another and experienced regimens of chemotherapy. I was pleased that when asked about these treatments, Mickelson did not hold back; he spoke meaningfully about how hard chemotherapy is. Too often, I now know, when we hear someone talk of chemotherapy some time after they have endured it, their words are tempered by the months or years of recovery that have passed. It sounds at worst like they wore a cast for a while and came away just fine.

Chemotherapy comes in many types and programs, but it is no patient's idea of a good time. In the hospital it made me pee incessantly and robbed me of my appetite almost immediately. I'll spare you some of the other effects, but with the radiation exacting its own pound of flesh, I had no interest in returning for round two of those daily chemo infusions. Even worse were the weeks following the chemo and radiation treatments. I slept all the time and didn't sleep at all. I'd feel well enough to sit at my computer and do my basic work right up until I didn't—which sometimes was no more than fifteen minutes later. I can honestly say that except for the days in the hospital, I never missed a day of work; but I did miss many hours, and I often had to reduce what I was doing to only the most essential tasks. I never feared that I wouldn't recover, but the waiting was punctuated with nausea and fatigue and difficulty eating. No, I will never again discount the harshness of chemotherapy, but I won't dwell on it either. That would be like a woman obsessing over the pain of her labor and seeing no joy in the child it brings.

For all the medical help I was receiving, another layer of support kept coming my way—out of the woodwork and out of the blue.

Just a week before my treatments were to begin, I received a phone call from a woman I had never met, though we had exchanged emails. She was a reader of the daily devotional I have been writing and editing since 2000, and she had sent encouragement through the years. Now she was calling because she heard from a mutual friend what I was facing. She and her husband, she said, had a house in Palo Alto they wanted to share with us. They lived elsewhere at this time of year, but they wanted to make the space available as we needed it. My wife's many years as a hospital nurse have supplied us with excellent insurance, and we would rely heavily on it as the bills added up to more than a million dollars by the time all the major work was done; but there were other expenses, not the least of which would have been lodging in an expensive part of California for the weeks of my hospitalization. Now Bob and Sue McCollum were offering hospitality to near strangers. Moreover, Sue is herself a cancer survivor, treated at Stanford, and the McCollums have made significant contributions to the radiation oncology department. In more ways than one, we were in her backyard, and we were being excessively blessed by their engagement. Through the years, Sue has built a support network called My Blue Dots, and she enlisted the women in her Bible study group in Southern California to pray for me, send notes and photos of encouragement, and stand with us.

The house in Palo Alto was always a blessing, but we lived three hours from Stanford and in the weeks when I had a 20-minute radiation treatment each day for five straight days, it made more sense to come home and return the next morning. I could go into my office if I felt up to it and sleep in my own bed. I tried as much as possible to continue coaching the high school golf team that I had led for ten years. If I could enlist a group of friends to step up, one or two a day, to drive with me to Stanford, the rides passed quickly. After a message on Facebook asking for this kind of help from among friends, people we saw regularly and those we had not seen in some time from our previous church offered to take a turn. The conversations kindled and rekindled took the repetition out of the drive. This also made it possible for Laura to continue taking shifts at the hospital a couple of days a week. And back in Fresno, my former pastor and long-time friend Brad Davis joined with some parents and my own dad to help coach the team. The number of helpers multiplied quickly.

The abundance of help also added up at the hospital. Each time I went for a stay, there were nurses and lab techs and medical teams that supported the surgeons and oncologists. I never properly appreciated the phlebotomists, whose typical visits came in the wee hours. They would open the door with a too loud "good morning," throw on the overhead lights so they could find the veins they needed, and do their work. Then they would glide out, leaving me to find my position of comfort again and try to snatch a couple more hours' sleep before the doctors showed up to see how I was doing. It was all part of the overall care, though, so those "vampires" were aiding the doctors too by giving them the information they needed to know if all was well.

During the first day of my first week in the hospital, though, I was introduced to a couple who would become especially dear. Carl had been there before me—he had come for his second round of chemo, while I was there for my first. It didn't take us long to compare notes and discover that we each had cancerous tumors in the neck and that we were each headed for surgery. The details weren't all the same, but they were enough that we each received a text that day. It was from Dr. Ganjoo, our common oncologist. She wanted to know, because she thought it would be helpful, if we wanted to meet this "other patient with a similar situation" who had checked in that day. She couldn't reveal more without our permission. We laughed and texted her back. Not only had we met, but we were roommates! Carl's beautiful optimism, his enjoyment of sports, his interest in our family, his sweet wife Francesca— this transplanted Aussie possessed all kinds of traits that enabled a great connection. In the ensuing year, Carl's medical challenges have proven to be far harder than mine, yet we exchange texts and arrange personal visits and I have watched him cling tenaciously to that optimistic perspective. He and Francesca have never left our prayer list.

WHEN THE CHEMOTHERAPY ENDED as we moved into May, I was thrashed. I brought the computer from my office home and fought hard to do the basics. Sometimes I would feel strong, get off the couch, and sit down to work, only to fall into nausea within a matter of minutes. Once, after several days of this ability to work for only fifteen and twenty minutes at a time, I barked at God. "Why, Lord, when I'm doing your work, can't you just let me be?" I have spoken many times about the name of God's people. We are Israel, those who wrestle with God, but all too often we present ourselves in our own strength as smooth-going Christians. *Nothing to see here. Move along.*

In Scripture, though, it started with Job and continued through the kings and prophets. They did not doubt God, but they were bold in questioning him. Where so many dismiss God over hard questions today, Job, Hannah, Moses, David, Elijah, Isaiah, and Jeremiah all looked at the troubles and injustices around them and said, in essence, "God who is allowing all this, tell me what you are doing!"

The answers aren't easy to find. I'm not sure that if God gave us the answers we think we want they would make sense to us anyway. I believe that these answers will one day come through quite clearly, or the questions will simply fall away. But I am for now locked into the finite mind of one living in a finite context. God's ways and thoughts are higher. I want them to be. To comprehend him would be to demote him—it can't be done.

One thing I could not do for even a couple of miles was

drive. The nausea would wipe me out. One day I made it to my office—two and a half miles—but when I got out of the car and tried to walk the thirty steps to my door, I couldn't get all the way there without going down to my knees. Another day my assistant showed up to find me laid out on the floor just waiting for the ill feelings to subside. So mostly I stayed home. Others drove me when they could (oddly, I was fine as a passenger). In mid-May, I went with a couple of my players to get in a practice round for a big tournament, and I tried to play with them. I managed two holes on the front nine and a couple more on the back. But I couldn't hit the ball half as far as I was used to and even driving the golf cart made me sick.

I only say all this because such experiences are common. The weeks following radiation and chemotherapy can be the hardest. Your body has been through things it wasn't designed to take. At the same time, the healthy body as God made it features stunning capabilities for immunity and recovery. Other than this tumor, I was healthy. I'd lost about ten percent of my body weight, and I was weakened, yes, but a comeback was not unexpected. It was just slow in coming.

This was the window during which my youngest son Josh graduated from college. A week after my radiation ended, we traveled to Southern California for the celebration. My oldest son and his wife flew in from Seattle, and their visit only made them witnesses to my unkind state. I left a family lunch to be sick in the bathroom. They stayed with me, though, during the ceremony, holed up in the hotel room and watching Josh walk via the internet. By the time we dropped Carson and Chelley off at the airport, I could hardly talk. I spent the next four hours laid out in the back seat as we drove home. I know all this rattled my daughter-in-law, whose spirit is beautifully tender, but this was my condition. I couldn't leave it, so I took it as it came. And sometimes it came with brutishness.

My surgery was scheduled and rescheduled, with a date finally locked in for July. In the middle of June, I had a pre-op appointment at Stanford. Laura traveled with me, which she wanted to do as often as she could. I deeply appreciated having her along for any number of marital reasons, but she was also my medical expert and advocate. She spoke the doctors' language and whenever she would hesitate to say that she was a nurse, I would speak up, because once this became known, the conversation would change. The providers at Stanford knew that she understood, and from her end there was an easing of anxiety when she knew more details about my care. What we also came to discover was that she and I would remember different things from our conversations with the doctors and our collective memory helped us both as we processed next steps—something that often doesn't happen until the hours after the actual appointment.

For this trip, I suggested that we stay the night closer to San Francisco and take in a Giants game. I arranged for a hotel room a couple of train stops from the stadium, and we made our way there. When it came time, we walked the two blocks to the station, a short trek but one that included a steep set of stairs. By the time we got to the station, I felt horrible. The nausea and weakness told me just one thing: *You should not be doing this.* Then the train came. We got on board and settled into a seat. When we arrived, we walked two more blocks to the stadium and rode the escalator to our level. We found our section and sunk into our chairs. I don't think I moved for the next three hours, other than to let others in and out. The game ended in a win for the Giants, but I don't think that's what cured me. Something did, though—the healing hand of God delivered on the cool bay air changed everything. When the game ended, we walked the long series of ramps down to street level and then back to the train. I felt fine. We ascended those steep steps on the other end and returned to the hotel room.

From that night forward, I felt like me for the next four weeks, right up to the surgery. I played golf a couple of times without any fatigue and enjoyed those early summer days like normal. A few weeks before I had asked a friend to help me with my yard—several guys offered—because I couldn't mow our tiny lawn without exhaustion. Now I could do all that work and all the work of the ministry, too. In the months I have now lived since those harshest days, I have said many times over that I have been shown many mercies though all this. Here was the first. A month of normalcy. And I know now that there are many, many sufferers out there who would love the same.

the ministering touch of Jesus

JULY 11. SURGERY DATE. This was the day we first thought would happen six months sooner.

Every necessary pre-op appointment at Stanford had taken place, including the one with the vascular surgeon. One thing looked certain: I would lose my carotid artery on one side. The tumor encased it and could not be removed without snipping the artery and grafting in a synthetic section. Carl had needed this procedure during his surgery, which by this time was several weeks past.

Late in the game, though, we received a call from Stanford. They had nearly forgotten that I needed basic physical clearance from my GP back home. Dr. Mu and I had not seen each other since that fateful day in December 2015. I made the required appointment to see him again the Thursday before surgery, which would come on a Monday. That week I was busy with one last task. I had agreed to preach at my home church that Sunday morning. This was the first of three sermons I would deliver between this mid-summer day and New Year's Day. All of them would be tinged with the experience of my year.

My treatments had led me to see anew the ministering actions of Jesus. We are not wrong to read and love Jesus' words. You may even own a Bible that highlights those words in red. One of the reasons we go back and back to the words of Jesus is because of their timelessness; they instruct us as well today as they did those first disciples when Jesus spoke them.

But let's consider those disciples for a moment. What they learned of Jesus was not just a litany of uttered precepts. They watched him do his thing, you might say. When he sent them out to heal and cast out demons, they went in the confidence of having seen what he himself had done. I became interested, sometimes fascinated, during the course of treatments in the way that doctors and nurses serve us—that is, how they minister to our physical bodies. This was not only a matter of words but of action. Few of these actions were monumental. Most were mundane and repetitive—just like, we might say, Jesus' washing of his disciples' feet. Many of these actions, especially when it came to healing, centered on his touch.

In Mark 5, Jesus was summoned by a desperate synagogue ruler whose daughter was gravely ill. Jesus agreed to return with the man, Jairus, to his house to minister to his daughter, but while they were on the way, some men came from the house and reported that the girl was no longer sick but had died. Jesus spoke important words next. He said to the ruler, "Do not fear, only believe." And they kept going until they arrived at the ruler's house and Jesus sent the mourners out, telling them that the girl was only asleep. Now we pick up the narrative in verse 40: "But he put them all outside and took the child's father and mother and those who were with him and went in where the child was. Taking her by the hand he said to her, '*Talitha cumi*,' which means, 'Little girl, I say to you, arise.' And immediately the girl got up and began walking (for she was twelve years of age), and they were immediately overcome with amazement."

Don't miss Jesus' tiny action in the midst of his life-restoring words. He took the girl by the hand. That is, he touched her. It is critical to understand that Jesus' touch was not necessary for healing. He healed others from afar, and in many of the healing accounts there is no reference to his touch. But we do know this: people desired the physical touch of Jesus.

The full account in Mark 5 tells us about the bleeding woman who touched Jesus while he was on his way to the house of the ruler. This woman said to herself, "If I just touch his clothes, I will be healed." And we know that when she touched him, not only was she healed, but Jesus instantly recognized that he had been touched—not brushed up against in the crowd, but purposefully touched with the effect that healing power went forth from him.

Look, too, at Mark 10: "And they were bringing children to him that he might touch them, and the disciples rebuked them. But when Jesus saw it, he was indignant and said to them, 'Let the children come to me; do not hinder them, for to such belongs the kingdom of God.'" These people understood a connection between the ministering love of Jesus and his touch. And Jesus responded favorably.

Touch remained significant in the ministry of the apostles. In Acts 6, those called as deacons were prayed over with the laying on of hands. In Acts 8, Peter and John laid their hands on the new Samaritan believers and they received the Holy Spirit. In Acts 13, Paul and Barnabas were commissioned with prayer and the laying on of hands. In Acts 28, Paul healed a man on the island of Malta, with prayer and the laying on of hands. We know from Paul's letters to Timothy that his protégé was called into ministry by Paul's own laying on of hands but also by the laying on of hands of the body of elders.

Touch is not magic—we cannot say it occurs in every instance of healing or commissioning or Holy Spirit imparting. It's not magic, but it's ministerial.

And so we return to my appointment with Dr. Mu. The purpose of this pre-op visit was to conduct a physical, so that he would attest that I was generally well enough to undergo the surgery. In a way, this is a ridiculous. Doctors were about to cut into my body and extract a tumor of still unverified nature from some of the more intricate regions of my anatomy. Not all surgeries are the same. Some occur daily, often multiple times, in hospitals around the world. A doctor might rightly say that you are well enough to withstand the rigors of a surgery like this. But my surgery? The only guarantees at this point were that it would take a long time, that cancer cells would be left, that my vagus nerve would be compromised (which could affect any number of things, including my speech), and that I would have a Gore-Tex line in place of my own natural carotid artery. If Dr. Mu could sign me off for a surgery like that, he would be doing so "only so far as he could."

But he went a step farther than that.

After checking off the required boxes and okaying me for surgery, he asked if he could pray for me. We had in our very limited doctor-patient experience established my line of work, so he felt comfortable in stepping forward now. Of course, I agreed, and he moved in closer to me, then asked if I minded if he held my hand. So there it is: two Christian men, one ministering to the other with the holiness of pure touch. And then he prayed a prayer so deferential to the sovereignty of God and so laced with the deep truths of Scripture that I couldn't help but think, *This man must be an elder in his church*. Maybe it was a silly thought, too closely connected to our understandings of the religious establishment, but I recognized this: not many men pray like that. They must carry a confidence in the God who sustains them and in what he can do, and they must be willing to bear the weight of responsible leadership. These are traits to which every believing man should aspire, but not so many possess them. Fewer still are willing to employ them in unfamiliar company. Dr. Mu dared. And in this way, he ministered to me as Jesus ministers—both by his words and by his actions, including the action of touch.

These of course were not the only prayers I received. I had family praying, friends old and new praying, readers of mine praying, and church friends praying praying. The outreach was overwhelming.

At the front of all these was my pastor, Ben Dosti, whose own prayers for me, every single time we met as elders, were for a complete healing. Ours is not a Pentecostal or even charismatic church by the common definitions, and Ben's own theological background is suspicious of some of the spiritual gifts these other churches emphasize, but when it came to my healing he was as bold as a miracle worker. We know what God can do in one's spirit; why should we doubt what he can do in our bodies? So Ben prayed without limits and without reservation. That day before my surgery, he called the congregation forward, as many as could get to the front, to surround Laura and me with their physical support by the laying on of hands and spiritual covering in prayer. We who had so often ministered in our lives were the objects of ministry. All those prayers as they were prayed in the weeks and months leading to this day lingered before the throne of God and echoed in his ears as I lay on the table the following day.

masters at work

THAT SUNDAY AFTERNOON, Laura and I climbed into the car and drove to Palo Alto. We were due at the hospital early the next morning, where I would be prepped for surgery and the tumor would come out.

As we sat at the McCollums' dinner table eating takeout, my phone rang. The number showed a Palo Alto area code, so I figured it was the hospital giving some final instructions or modifying the plan. Instead, I was surprised to hear Dr. Holsinger announce himself. Our pre-meal prayers had included entreaties that this man and his colleagues would be guided throughout the surgery. I couldn't help but say, "We were just praying for you." He offered me some assurances that the team had been reviewing my case through the weekend and they were ready to go. Nothing too clinical and not very long. A perfect call for the moment.

I slept fine that night, though it didn't matter. My body would be asleep for hours the next day.

If this book is about all the people God provided for my help, I could fill it with the parade of people who helped me in the first three hours of that Monday morning, starting with the two people who checked me in and the nurse who walked me back to pre-op and gave me instructions for changing into my surgical gown. Members of Dr. Holsinger's team—residents and fellows—came by, as did those from Dr. Berry's team and also from the vascular surgeon, Dr. Matthew Mell. These men checked in personally, too, of course.

Then there were the anesthesiologists. Laura works with these doctors daily in her role at the children's hospital, so her question many weeks before for Dr. Berry had been about his choice in anesthesiologists. His answer was unequivocal: "I only work with the best." Part of that is a confidence-giving tactic, sure, but it doesn't mean you don't like to hear it! Anesthesiology is a strange business, at least in the interaction between doctor and patient. They introduce themselves just ahead of the surgery, then do everything they can to kindly assure you that everything will be okay while at the same time deeply piercing your skin and veins for a "good poke." After that, you may see them again for a matter of moments on the operating table. At least that's the way it was for me. Moments. After sliding over from my gurney, I cannot say I lay on the table for more than a ten-count before I was gone. Somehow, though, ahead of all this, the two men who controlled my wakefulness (and lack of it) that day secured my confidence. One of them, a big but entirely disarming man looked at me closely in the prep room and asked, "Are you a praying man?" Between his question and his response to my answer—"So am I"—we knew we were on the same page, where faith intertwined with medicine.

After every layer of checking and double checking, Laura and I had a chance to kiss goodbye, then I was rolled to surgery and she went out to wait.

For all I can speak to about what happened to me in those many months, my report from the next few hours is severely lacking in firsthand references. Laura could tell me what she and my parents and my sons Daniel and Josh did to while away the long hours, and the doctors could tell us what went on in the operating room, where as many as twenty different people came and went while I remained quiet and prone.

But for all this, the man in the middle, Dr. Chris Holsinger, was made to wait.

The doctors anticipated a ten-hour surgery. In from the back to free the tumor atop and above the lungs, then an incision in the neck to remove the tumor from its threatening berth. Dr. Berry scalpeled through the skin and thin muscle of my back, then used a rib separator to give him room to work. But that work was met with more difficult resistance than expected and two hours dragged to four, five, six. As the seventh hour approached, a decision had to be made. If Dr. Holsinger—who had scrubbed twice in preparing to begin his procedures—set in now, and Dr. Mell intervened to do his part with my carotid artery, we were looking at twelve to fourteen hours or more. No one was prepared for that.

Only later, when I was recovering in my hospital room, would Dr. Holsinger tell us that something came over him at that point. He could sense that the surgery was not supposed to go ahead. Not then. For me, this was his way of telling me, whether he meant to or not, that the Spirit of God had governed the decisions of the lead surgeon that day. One of the best in world, still Dr. Holsinger had not gotten ahead of himself. He listened to what he could not really hear. The rest of the operation would have to wait five weeks. We—and especially Laura—were going to have to go through it all again. But we knew that was best.

The greatest challenge in the aftermath of that first surgery remains to this day. The vagus nerve runs a circuit from the brain to the colon, affecting the function of most everything from the vocal cords to the heart and lungs to the digestive tract. Compromise this path and a number of changes can result. In my case, a compromise was expected with all the intricate moves around the structures of my neck. But it came earlier, with my left vocal cord paying the price of paralysis. The day-to-day effect means some swallowing difficulty and coughing, but the most notable change occurred in my voice. It is deeper, thinner, and lacks volume to carry past even slight ambient noise. In a quiet room, one on one, you might just think me a long-time smoker. But at church or in a restaurant, I'll lean in to help you out by speaking into your ear or face up to you so you have the added advantage of reading my lips. Laura and I have learned to be more intimate when we go out to dinner; we sit on the same side of the table now! Public speaking has almost always been a significant part of my life, and thanks to microphones it still can be. Though I am not as faithful in it as I would like to be, I haven't stopped praying for healing. Blind Bartimaeus cried out to Jesus. So can I. Beyond that, God will do what he will do.

- - -

FIVE WEEKS LATER, ON AUGUST 15, we returned. Now Dr. Holsinger could have his fun. That may sound like I am jesting, but the day I emerged from post-op ICU and could make sense of what people were saying to me, he came to my room and told me it was a "pleasure and a privilege" to do my surgery. I thought, *Here is a person at the height of his profession being given a chance to face a true challenge*—like Jack Nicklaus or Tiger Woods putting their skills to the test against a course brilliantly and sternly designed. Or, to reference the kind of show my wife and I like to watch, like Bobby Flay in the midst of a throwdown. But in neither of those cases do the experts have someone's life in their hands. Dr. Holsinger had mine.

We were of course used to the routine now. Show up early, having eaten nothing, change into my gown, receive the various probes and pokes, and wait to be rolled away. The nurses were different this time and the anesthesiologists, too. More helpers. The numbers just kept accumulating.

When I came to the operating room, I may have survived an extra second or two before the drip put me out—long enough to have an anti-sore patch placed on my tailbone and to lay back on the table. See ya. In the next ten hours, I would receive an incision running from just beneath my left ear lobe, under my chin and across my throat, then straight down my chest like a patient in open-heart surgery.

While Dr. Berry still had work to do inside my chest wall, Dr. Holsinger's work would take centerstage this time—but for the part where Dr. Mell would step in to graft the Gore-Tex section into my carotid artery. Except this never happened. As he described it to us later, when it came time to snip the carotid on either end of the tumor, Dr. Holsinger hesitated. In the classic question of curiosity, he thought, *Why not?* Then he began to slice away the tumor little by little, "filleting it," he said, until it fell away from the artery. I'm not given to hyperbole myself, so I don't want to accuse another of it; that's why I continue to think it a pretty big deal that Dr. Holsinger told us at a follow-up appointment that this was a highlight of his career.

Can you really say whether one doctor or another is one of the world's top surgeons? When you get to the very best, there's no point in ranking them. If a surgeon saves your life—or at least makes it significantly better or meaningfully longer—he or she is as good as you'll ever need, whether doing their work at Stanford Medical Center or an emergency room in a remote corner of Canada. No one ever said this surgery of mine was going to be easy, and there was a reason the ENT doctor in Fresno referred me on. Compromises and sacrifices were made in order for the most important goal to be accomplished. These many months later I still have numbness in my shoulder and chest and my swallowing can turn to a nasty fit of coughing if everything isn't quite right going down. But the "guarantee," the biggest risk for complication after my surgery—that my carotid would come out—didn't materialize. As I've said, I have spoken repeatedly to friends and family of the many mercies I received in 2016. That my carotid artery is still in its "factory packaging"—that was my miracle.

Ten hours of surgery is a breeze for the patient, at least when it comes to conscious awareness. Outside Laura waited. She didn't wait alone. I had adamantly encouraged my youngest son to keep travel plans he had to Hawaii. But my parents were there, my middle son Daniel, my sister Kendra, and our dear friends Marty and Barbara Jacobus. Marty is the CEO of the ministry with which I have served for 17 years, Links Players. He and his wife have their own gut-wrenching and gorgeous stories of widowhood and remarriage, and also of their own daunting medical issues. Like almost no one we know, this couple understands major illness, hospitals, surgeries, and waiting to see what God will do when you are so far out of your comfort zone you might as well be floating without a lifeline in outer space. Now they came, only to sit with Laura and keep her talking when she needed conversation but keep their distance when she just needed to be still and know God is God. Can I just say: If you don't have friends like this, get them! You may not think you need them now, but you will someday. For all the helpers God will give you, his greatest provision for you beyond salvation will be friends like this. You don't need many, maybe only one or two. But they will be there, sticking closer when you most need them.

the provision of people

FOR ONE OF THOSE REASONS that is inexplicable to us but very much known to God, in the year or so leading up to my diagnosis, I found myself thanking God often for his provision. In this, I mean the typical things we speak of when reflecting on God's provision: food, shelter, a job—the basics. I have never been a fan of those who pray without restraint when it comes to saying "grace," that prayer before a meal. In the natural realm, I can't shake the thought that this carefully prepared food is growing cold in those extended minutes of a prayer. If you want to hold a vigil, that's fine. But maybe another time is better. I think Jesus felt the same. Several times in the Gospels, we read of him "giving thanks" before a meal. That's it. "Giving thanks." Not lifting up the infirmed masses and interceding for revival. Doubtless, Jesus prayed through the night for things like these, but he did not pray this way before a meal. So my prayers of thanks for provision were generally quick and tidy.

Then came the walk through cancer of which I have already told you. And in reflecting on all the circumstances comprising that year, I began to see one thing in common through all the help I received: people. Whether they were

39

praying people or hospitable people or doctors, nurses, techs or others in the medical community, God brought us people to provide his care for us. Some were friends, others strangers; all were part of God's design and timing. This has been true through the ages.

We are fond in the community of faith of saying that God will never leave us alone. What we rarely recognize, however, is that his presence is continually spelled out through people. Specifically prepared people arrive in perfect time. This is not an accident. It is a display of God's sovereign hand.

In the Old Testament book of 1 Samuel, we are introduced to two men who were not ignorant of the way God had brought them together. In God's initial establishment of Saul as king, his son Jonathan should have one day been king. Instead, with Saul's disdain for obedience, his line was removed from the throne and a shepherd named David was anointed to replace him. If ever two men should not have been close, it was Jonathan and David. But God had given Jonathan a humble and faithful heart. With it, he recognized the sins of his father and the righteousness of David. So Jonathan threw all the support he could behind his friend.

In 1 Samuel 30, David found himself in a dreadful place: home. In those days, David and his men had established residence for their families in Ziklag. Their wives and children lived there at a time when David's army found a place in assisting Achish, the king of Gath. A disagreement arose between Achish and the leaders of the Philistines, and David was dismissed, along with all his men. This was only the beginning of the bad news. When these men returned home, they found that Ziklag had been raided by the Amalekites. The men's wives were gone, taken captive, along with everyone else in the town, both "great and small." The city itself had been burned.

Among the men, the emotion was great. We are told that they "wept until they had no more strength to weep." But as so often happens among human beings, our sorrows must come with someone to blame. In this case, the finger was pointed at David. In verse 6, we find this:

David was greatly distressed, for the people spoke of stoning him, because all the people were bitter in soul, each for his sons and daughters.

DAVID HAD EVERY REASON to feel alone in this hour. His family was gone, and now his own life was in danger. But the verse is not over (nor the story). Here is what we read next: "But David strengthened himself in the LORD his God." This makes perfect sense. When you're alone, find a friend in Jesus. Go to God. And sure enough, when David consulted of the LORD, he received the instruction he needed to go forward and find his family.

Before we go on, however, let's take a look back, to 1 Samuel 23. Here David was hiding from Saul, who was pursuing him and looking to end David's life. Jonathan, we are told, went to David at Horesh and "helped him find strength in God."

We might stop here and say that this is what friends do for one another. They support each other in dark times. But Jonathan came at risk of his own life, and rather than playing the hero, he trained David's focus in God's direction. This was training David would need when the threat was even nearer, when his fiercest supporters were ready to turn on him.

But the story goes on. When David consulted with the LORD, God assured him that he would succeed if he pursued the Amalekites. His men took heart at this and went with David to find their wives and children. But as the chase went on, some the men became tired and were left behind. Those who continued had no certain trail until they came upon an Egyptian, abandoned to die in the desert. They fed the man and asked him what he was doing alone in the wasteland. He explained that he had been a slave of an Amalekite who had forsaken him when he had fallen ill three days prior. David asked the now-revived man if he could lead them to the Amalekites, and in exchange for safety the Egyptian did so. When David's men found the Amalekites, they succeeded in battle and recovered their wives, children, and household goods.

Now recognize the difference between Jonathan and the Egyptian. The former was a dear friend, the latter a complete stranger. Yet both had significant roles to play in assisting David at critical times. This is the nature of God's provision of people. We must keep our eyes open for it at all times, never pre-judging, for we cannot know for sure ahead of time whom God will use to come to our aid.

Though it was not my intended end of my original teaching on this matter, a friend eager to study and eager to put her faith into action came to me a week later and said her entire view of others had changed that week. Now she was looking to see whom God was sending her way. She was seeing the Lord's hand in the people who crossed her path—wherever she went. Sometimes they were put there for her to help them, but it was also quite possible that God had sent them to help her, and she didn't want to miss it.

With this understanding that God's assistance may come from any direction, I want to show you the ways God may send people to you. There are seven of them that I will touch on here. You may find more.

People to help you

First, God provides people to help us. At Stanford, I had five doctors working together to remove my tumor and effectively save my life: an oncologist, a radiologist, a vascular surgeon, a thoracic surgeon, and a head & neck surgeon. I did not know any of these people, of course. I was referred by my primary care doctor to a local ENT physician then on to the head & neck surgeon at Stanford. In addition to being one of the top surgeons of his type in the world, Dr. Holsinger is one of the most personable people on the planet and a man who understands faith. He could have in pride chosen to function on his own. But I'll tell you this: we never saw him alone. He was himself a stunning example of one who relied on the help of others. Always, there were a physician's assistant and a nurse coordinator and residents and fellows and students and visiting doctors hanging around. He worked with them and the other doctors on the tumor board to keep up the conversation about my case and my care.

Again, this was not accident or coincidence. At one point we were asked by an assistant, "How did you get to Stanford?" We told her that it was a direct referral from the ENT doctor in Fresno to Dr. Holsinger. She replied, "That's wonderful. So many people go here and there and another place and another place before they get to us, and by the time they get here, we say, 'If only you'd gotten here sooner.'" I had an extremely unusual case that required extremely specialized help. I even said to Dr. Holsinger, thinking here of the Lord's precise provision: "I was not referred to you; you were referred to me."

We can ask God for help of every kind, and it may come, as we've noted, from unexpected directions or from people we have not previously known. But we can also ask those he has already given to us in the family of faith. This is what Paul did when he urged Timothy: "Do your best to come to me soon… When you come, bring the cloak that I left with Carpus at Troas, also the books, and above all the parchments" (2 Timothy 4:9, 13). The help we receive can be so down-to-earth practical that we don't recognize it as God's provision. This is our loss, for every time we thank him we are in reality worshiping him. Don't hesitate to ask God for help and don't fail to thank him. We want to be like the one who returned to Jesus, eager to show him our gratitude for the way he has helped us.

People to guide you

Second, God will give you guides. This is what the deserted Egyptian became for David and his men as they attempted to locate the Amalekites. When you travel in foreign countries, you normally hire a guide. You do this for one reason: the guide knows what you do not. And the guide knows what you do not because the guide has been here before, often many times. With this knowledge and experience, they can show you the way. A good guide in a foreign country is worth far more than a map. These guides have their connections, for meals, for shops, and most importantly for safety.

I found in the year of my cancer that some of the best provision God gave me came from people who had been there before me. In my small home church of just 200 people, there were two who had been to Stanford ahead of me for cancer treatments. One of these actually had a tumor removed from her neck in a procedure very similar to mine. Since, we have added a fourth Stanford cancer patient. We have compared notes, asked each other questions, and been guides for one another, even crossing paths those three hours from home when our appointments have lined up. It sure is nice to see a familiar face when the slog of treatments grows old. I'd go so far as to call it God's treat!

I do not want to fail to mention, though, that again God can provide the most unexpected people. When I met Carl as my roommate during my first hospitalization, he was enduring his second hospital go-around. I have to confess that when it was time for my second go-around, I was anything but excited. But here came Carl, who not only could tell me what to expect when it came to treatment, but tell me what to order off the menu and where to go to get a better view. He was friendly with my son and friendly with my parents. Carl's guidance was a major encouragement. One more thing: Carl is a huge soccer fan. He's a founding member of the fan club of the San Francisco Deltas. The Deltas love Carl, too, and they reached out to this superfan by giving him penalty cards. Carl would hand these out to other patients and declare, "Give a red card to cancer." He was not just a guide but a strong encourager; now I am doing all I can to be his encourager, too, as Carl's fight has been much greater than mine.

If what you need is a guide to show you the way—not so much as one brilliantly trained but as one who "knows the streets" you will be walking—ask the Lord. He can give you such a guide, among those you know and those you don't.

People to pray for you

Third, see how God provides people to pray for you. I'm going to be open right here. I am not a fan of giant prayer circles. I do not see anywhere in Scripture where the result of a prayer comes by way of how many people are praying. Certainly I don't see that our prayers are more favorably answered if we post our needs far and wide on social media. I don't think it works that way.

But I will tell you that I am in no way resistant to prayer. I have already mentioned that *every single time* we prayed together as elders in our church for what was going on in my body, our senior pastor prayed boldly for miracles, and specifically for the miracle of complete healing—as in, "Just make the tumor disappear, Lord." We believe that God will acts as he wills. But we do not see in Scripture examples of mealy-mouthed, waffling prayers: "Well, you know, God, what I would really like is for this amazing thing to happen, but it's your will and all that, so if you're thinking something different I'll live with it, I guess..." Are you kidding? James essentially said, "Don't you dare pray like that!" Look at James 1: "If any of you lacks wisdom, let him ask God, who gives generously to all without reproach, and it will be given him. But let him ask in faith, with no doubting, for the one who doubts is like a wave of the sea that is driven and tossed by the wind. For that person must not suppose that he will receive anything from the Lord; he is a double-minded man, unstable in all his ways." The context there starts specific to wisdom, but it ends with "anything." It's a principle for all prayer, like Jesus' words in John 14: "Whatever you ask in my name, this I will do, that the Father may be glorified in the Son. If you ask me anything in my name, I will do it."

Guess what? You're going to mess up. The people who are praying for you are going to mess up. You're going to pray selfishly, or they're going to ask for things that God has no intention of answering according to the way they are asking. God can sort all that out. Never pray fearfully; pray faithfully. Do we or do we not believe that Jesus meant what he said? The answer to this question is vital, because people will come alongside you in prayer—whether for healing if you are sick or discernment if you are making a difficult decision or peace if the circumstances of your life are tumultuous—and they are doing so because they believe God can intervene. What a shame it would be if all those people believed for me and I did not believe with them!

Here is what happened for us: People started praying. And they started asking others to pray, even though this isn't what we in our privacy thought we wanted. We can laugh about this now. We can laugh about it because one of my colleagues said, "You know, the prayer of a righteous person is powerful and effective. The more people praying, the better chance there is that one of them is righteous!" He was kidding. Maybe. But here's what else we can do about all these pray-ers praying all these prayers. We can rejoice that God provided people to pray for us from among the expected and from among the unexpected. In the last days before my first surgery, I had a Catholic friend tell me that he would light every candle at his church for me and I had a Mormon neighbor tell me she had added me to the prayer list at the temple. I'm not going to get into the theology of all that. What I am going to say is that Laura and I were led to ask God to answer these prayers for one reason: that the people who were praying would see that he is at work. We wanted people of great faith to become people of greater faith, and we wanted people of little faith to see their faith enlarged to the size of a mustard seed (because in God's economy, a mustard seed is really big!).

I believe that so much of what happened in my favor happened because people were praying. But more than that I believe that it happened so that those who prayed would see the wonder of God and continue to call on his name. Ask God to surround you with praying people. Ask him to answer their prayers for his own glory. Then look for what God does through the prayers of the people he provides.

People to care for you

Fourth, I found that God gave me people to care for me. In some ways this is similar to people who can help you, but let me explain a difference. The people who can help are often specially equipped to do so, as my doctors were. When my car breaks down, I look for help from a mechanic. When I don't know how to do a spreadsheet function, I Google the problem and watch one of the experts on the internet walk me through it. But care is so much simpler. It is something almost anyone can do, and yet those people have to be available and willing.

By the time my second trip to the hospital for chemo came around, I was having severe pain while swallowing. Eating pretty much anything off the hospital menu was out of the question. So Laura and I had a morning routine, where I would text her the flavor and size of Jamba Juice I wanted, and she would stop on the way to the hospital and pick one up. That's how simple this can be. But it's also out-of-the-way, on-someone-else's-timetable sort of simple, so not everybody is available and willing.

I have already told you about the biggest blessing of care we received: the hospitality of people we did not know offering us their house in Palo Alto as we needed it during hospitalization and treatments. This started with a phone call about a week before I went into the hospital. I told our hostess after my first hospital stay that I was blown away when I considered the web of sovereign connections, going back to my youth, that God had woven in order for the two of our paths to ever cross—but she still had to wake up that morning and say to herself, "I'm going to call Jeff and offer him our house." God provided care through a willing couple.

There are enough available passages to not include the Parable of the Good Samaritan in this little book, but that would be to ignore some of the best language of care we can find in Scripture. Look:

> But a Samaritan, as he journeyed, came to where he was, and when he saw him, he had compassion. He went to him and bound up his wounds, pouring on oil and wine. Then he set him on his own animal and brought

him to an inn and took care of him. And the next day he took out two denarii and gave them to the innkeeper, saying, 'Take care of him, and whatever more you spend, I will repay you when I come back.' Which of these three (including the Pharisee and the teacher of the law), do you think, proved to be a neighbor to the man who fell among the robbers?" He said, "The one who showed him mercy." (Luke 10:33-37)

If you think in mercy, you'll act in care. That's what God provided for me—merciful people who recognized that I was not in those days my usual self and that I needed little acts of caring to get through it. Depending on your circumstances, you may need experts to help you, but just as often you'll need people to provide simple, available care. You can ask God for this, too.

People to be with you
Fifth, there are the people to be with you. In many ways, having people with you is a subset of care. Sometimes we just need people to spend time with us, to come when no one else is coming. Laura was there; so were my parents—these I expected and greatly appreciated. But my sons and my sister came far out of the way. A church friend was working a project nearby and took the time to see me in the hospital. There were others traveling in the area who knew I was there and had a chance to drop in. The drivers who helped us go back and forth between Stanford nearly 30 times in two months helped make for a much better day each time, simply because they were present. Most of them wanted not only to drive but to talk and encourage us and pray. In this way, the people by themselves were the provision of God to us.

We know the names of at least five different people (Silas,

Andronicus, Junias, Aristarchus, and Epaphras) who shared prison cells with the apostle Paul. With Silas, Paul sang worship songs. Of the others, he spoke very warmly. A first century jail cell was even worse than a 21st century hospital room, yet Paul found the blessing of provision even here, as God sent others to join him in his trial.

What you may need God to provide right now is simply someone to visit. Ask him, then see how he provides.

People to understand you
Sixth, God will give you people who understand you and your circumstances. One of the most significant passages in Scripture for recognizing the way God forges a heart-to-heart relationship with us is found in Hebrews 4:15-16: "For we do not have a high priest who is unable to sympathize with our weaknesses, but one who in every respect has been tempted as we are, yet without sin. Let us then with confidence draw near to the throne of grace, that we may receive mercy and find grace to help in time of need."

Jesus can sympathize, Jesus can render mercy so well, because he has faced just what we have faced. He gets it. He gets us. And sometimes he gives us people who get us.

Earlier I mentioned my colleague Marty Jacobus, a dear partner in ministry. Let me tell you more of his story. Seven years ago, Marty lost his wife Jenny after a long battle with cancer in La Quinta, California, which is far down in the southern desert. About that same time a woman named Barbara Meyer, living up in Ukiah, well north of San Francisco, lost her husband David to pancreatic cancer. To make a long story short, these two, Marty and Barbara, were introduced to one another and married five years ago. Now here's the first thing: Barbara knew she wanted to marry only someone who had been widowed, someone who understood the grueling struggle. She found this in Marty. And here's the second thing: Barbara herself was diagnosed in 2015 with breast cancer. She has been undergoing treatment and after-treatment. Through this, Marty and Barbara's understanding deepened all the more. And here's the third thing: they have given that understanding as a gift to us. When Marty tells me he is praying for me, I know that he knows just what all this treatment is like for me and what all this emotional weight is like for Laura. And here's the fourth thing: Oh, the price Marty and Barbara have had to pay in order to minister to us like this! That's a very potent sovereignty God has wrought, both coming and going. For them, painfully potent; for us, mercifully so.

People for me to pray for
This seventh consideration may be the most surprising aspect of God's provision of people, for in it the tables turn. God may give you people to minister to in order to relieve you of the self-focus that can become so burdensome in times of difficulty.

Before I was diagnosed with cancer, others I knew who had received such news were few, and usually I did not know them well. But from the day I was diagnosed and going forward through the next eighteen months to the conclusion of this book, people I knew well and often was already ministering to were told they had cancer. There were six in the first nine months alone. Then another. And another. I was pressed into more urgent prayer—something I now did as someone who personally understood the anxieties and procedures of both the patients and the caregivers.

If praying is good for you all the time, it is really good for you when you need to get your eyes off your own circumstances. And it is really good for you when you know that other people have needs like yours and you are able to care and understand. What did Paul say of the body of Christ? "If one part suffers, every part suffers with it; if one part is honored, every part rejoices with it" (1 Corinthians 12:26). We need to know one another's hardest roads. And we need to pray for one another. You may even need to ask the Lord to give you people to pray for! We should all the time be building up our relationship with Jesus in prayer. That can happen in praying for ourselves. But this is Jesus, who said, "Love your neighbor as yourself." This is Jesus, who said, "Love your enemies and pray for those who persecute you."

Just like care, prayer can require availability and willingness. Intercessory prayer can carry real weight. You may be bearing people to Jesus on your spiritual back. But you are doing so for the very reason that in their weakness they cannot carry themselves. Caregivers have to be able to get up and get out, but prayer-givers can do their work from anywhere.

the ultimate person of provision

NO DOUBT, IT WOULD BE POSSIBLE to walk away from a book like this and think to yourself, *That was a bunch of good words about a bunch of good people. And I get that God would send these people to us. But what about God himself? Isn't he the one we really need?*

The answer is a resounding *yes*! But here is what is so stunning: when God gave himself to us, he came as a person. We call this the incarnation—God coming in the flesh to offer us the only thing that saves.

God, as the man Jesus of Nazareth, was born in rough conditions in Bethlehem, a shepherd's town outside of Jerusalem. He was laid in a manger, the Lamb among the sheep. He got lost as a boy, grew up in stature. He was trained in his father's carpenter shop, with sawdust in the hairs of his arms. He studied and memorized the Scriptures, just as his Jewish friends did. He attended weddings and funerals and Sabbaths in the synagogue. He visited the sick. He told stories and challenged theologians and rich men. He cooked fish on a beach and broke bread around a common table. In every way he was a man. Which means he was also disliked by others. Men hated his teaching and plotted his death. He was betrayed and brought to trial, scourged and led out to die. At Calvary, he was transfixed to the cross and in the end he gave up his spirit with the words, "It is finished." His work. And his fleshly life.

In the Old Testament, God also gave men to be intermediaries. They were the priests, who year upon year went to the altar on behalf of the people, making atonement for their sins by the blood of goats and calves.

But, we are told, Jesus entered the Holy of Holies "not by means of the blood of goats and calves but by means of his own blood, thus securing an eternal redemption" (Hebrews 9:12). The economy of God, mysterious in its design, says this: "Without the shedding of blood there is no forgiveness" (Hebrews 9:22). A spirit has no blood to shed. By coming as the man Jesus, born to be the Messiah, the Saving One, God could make for us the very atonement he required. I don't know why he chose this method, but I know that he fulfilled it.

In Scripture's closing book, Revelation, again and again Jesus is referred to as the Lamb. It is the Lamb who was slain. It is the Lamb by whose blood the accuser of the people of God was overcome. It is the Lamb whose shed blood makes the stained robes of the enduring believers white. It is the Lamb who is worshipped, over and over, by thousands and thousands. It is the Lamb. The same Lamb about whom John the Baptist, in flesh and blood looking at the man Jesus in flesh and blood, said, "Behold, the Lamb of God who takes away the sin of the world" (John 1:29).

I can stand as one healed today and tell you that God will send the people you need in your life. And while I cannot tell you just whom he will send, I can tell you that he has already sent the one you need for salvation. He is the expected one— the Messiah. And yet he is also the unexpected one, who had no interest in earthly thrones or the adulation of men. He is the one who has helped you in a way no one else can, bearing your sin on the cross. He *loves* you, *cares* for you, *attends* to you, *understands* you, *intercedes* for you, and *calls* you to be his own. "Come to me," he says, "all who labor and are heavy laden, and I will give you rest. Take my yoke upon you, and learn from me, for I am gentle and lowly in heart, and you will find rest for your souls" (Matthew 11:28-29).

In the context of historically orthodox Christianity, we often speak of the gospel, or the good news of salvation in Christ. That gospel begins with bad news—that we are sinners unable to find our lost selves and in desperate need of a Savior. But it ends with overwhelmingly wonderful news—that God has made a way through his Son Jesus to erase our sin's indictment against us and bring us into the present and future kingdom of the ruler of all. I have tried in recent months to reduce this gospel to its simplest expression. I think this is it: *I can't. God can.* That God steps in and helps when we can in no way help ourselves is the most meaningful truth in the universe. What is remarkable is that he has done so through a man of flesh and blood, Jesus.

If you are asking for God's provision, he will repeatedly give it to you through people. And if you are asking for God's ultimate provision, the salvation of your soul unto eternal life, he gives that through a person too. All you must do is believe it. Don't worry that your faith is small today; God's provision is as big and as complete as you will ever need.

the help you need

THEOLOGY IS NOT ENOUGH. We can be taught things about God that we affirm and even believe, but we do not act on them. This inaction is to our great detriment.

For five years in the first decade of the 2000s, I pastored a small church where I had already spent the previous 15 years with my wife and sons. We had a dear man in our church who was knowledgeable and generous. He was a favorite with me and with our people. But he also had severe diabetes and an infection developed in his feet. One day I received a call from his sister to tell me he had died. I was in shock; I had no idea he was so sick. But here's what broke my heart: he had told his sister he wasn't telling us at the church about his illness because he thought we were too faithless a people to help him. Maybe he was right—and that would be heartbreaking in another way. But we never had the chance to pray, never had the chance to help, because we were never asked. We may not have had the gift of faith among us, but I know we had the gift of helps. I would have loved the chance for this body of believers to come around him. Though we closed the church in 2009, I still watch those people pray for one another and help one another. Some of them were there to help me in my cancer year, seven years later. They certainly would have helped this man had he just asked.

Many people are quick to say that we must go to God for help. That's what this book has been saying all along. But sadly, there are many who also believe that they don't need the church to go to God. They are partly right. They can pray to God without the church. But what is more completely true is that God has designed us to live in the fellowship of the body of Christ—that is, he has given us the church to be the answer to many of our prayers. And the church is people. When you are committed not only to Jesus but to Jesus' people in local fellowship, an entire world of help is opened up to you. God's provision of help can come in the miraculous moment, but it more often comes through the common assistance of his people, or even through the special provision of people who have been uniquely and spiritually gifted by God to help you. God's people in the church depend on God for the heart and skills that can help you, just as you depend on God to answer your cry for help—and so he brings us together in his sovereign provision.

So why do we resist asking for help? The easy answer is pride. When we ask another for help, we are admitting that we are not smart enough or strong enough or healthy enough or prepared enough. We are lacking and we know it. But if we can just keep this little secret to ourselves, then we won't lose the respect of others.

Pride like this can keep us from asking for practical help. That's bad enough. Worse still, however, is that it can keep us from seeking spiritual help. We are people prone to temptation and thus to sin. Left to our own devices, we choose spiritually damaging options, even when we can clearly see the various possible consequences. We think wrong thoughts, believe wrong "truths," say wrong things, and do wrong things.

It's that comprehensive. When you fall out of regular, committed fellowship and the mutual ministry it provides, you walk away from God's provision for your soul. I hope you can see the danger in this.

Let me supply you with four good things you can ask your believing friends with whom you share fellowship to do for you. Remember, you're not asking them because God can't help you; you're asking them because God has already given them to you to help you.

Ask a friend to preach to you

You have perhaps heard the expression, "Preach the gospel to yourself every day." This is good… if you remember the truths of the gospel… if your mind isn't prone to lesser thoughts… if you're not too tired when you get home from work. Do you see how we can make excuses for not doing what is good for us? But if we ask someone we trust to preach to us, when we give them permission to speak the words we need to hear, they can call and say, "You need to hear this, so here goes."

There is a second reason you need the gospel rightly and repeatedly preached to you: because others will come falsely and frequently with words that are not the gospel. This happened to the Galatian church and their case study is a tragic one. They had abandoned what had been preached to them, falling into legalism. It was into this context that Paul wrote these words to them: "But even if we or an angel from heaven should preach to you a gospel contrary to the one we preached to you, let him be accursed" (Galatians 1:8).

Let's break this down. One: preaching is to be an active part of our lives—most usually as the recipients of preaching. And two: the preaching that must not be compromised is the preaching of the gospel. Again, plenty of other preaching will come your way, but much of it may not be good for you at all.

Now let's consider how we might test this. The Greek for preach is probably not exactly what you're thinking. You may be thinking—because we often say, "Preach it!" in a demonstrative tone—that preaching is giving someone spiritual what-for. It's calling someone on the carpet. But the Greek for preach is *euaggelizō*, which means first and foremost and in almost every context "to bring good news, to bear good tidings." We err when we think of preaching as something akin to admonishing rather than something akin to evangelizing. You, friend, need to hear the good news of salvation by God's grace through the death and resurrection of Christ—and you need a friend to give it to you regularly.

Now you may ask, "Why not just show up to church and listen to my pastor preach each week? Doesn't that do the trick?" It starts the trick, but when you invite a friend to preach the gospel to you, you are doing so on the basis of their personal knowledge of what tempts and tests you. Hopefully, they have learned the gospel well from your pastor (or theirs) and other biblical teachers and they can help you apply the gospel to your specific life.

Some of us are more prone to legalism. These people are like the Galatians, thinking they need to add to the work of Christ by works of their own. Others are more prone to what is called antinomianism. This second group of people are like some of the Romans, who discounted the price paid by Christ and used his grace as an excuse to go on sinning. Where are you apt to fall out of balance? Your friend who preaches the gospel to you will know. He or she will spot your typical signs of wandering and call you back to the place of right understanding and free but righteous living.

They will do this by preaching to you the fullness of the gospel. First, that your natural person is a slave to sin. And the consequence of that sin, when left unremedied, is death. If you do not come to Jesus in this life, you will not live with him in the next. Now, you may say, "That doesn't sound like good news to me." No, that is only the harsh news that sets up the good news. But if you don't know your need, you won't seek a solution; you won't seek a Savior. And so the full preaching of the gospel continues. There is Jesus, mighty to save, and willing. The blood of his crucifixion is the atoning agent, the remedy. It washes away our sin. It brings freedom from sin's grip. It empowers us to live as spiritual people. When this is the gospel you hear preached to you, you recognize in it the call away from unrighteousness and the impetus for righteous living that pleases and honors the King; you recognize in it that all your good works amount to nothing because they cannot stand up to his glorious work for you. You'll stop trying to save yourself with religion and start serving a Savior who loves you so much that he bore the weight of your sin on a criminal's cross.

That, friends, is the gospel. And it is what you need to have preached to you, so that you will be daily reminded that you are alive in Christ and living for him.

Ask a friend to pray for you

The second kind of help you need to ask for is prayer.

You have likely heard of several ways to express yourself in prayer. Sometimes you will hear this outlined as A-C-T-S: Adoration, Confession, Thanksgiving, Supplication. The "S" in that outline, Supplication, means to ask for things. A supplicant is someone who asks respectfully for something from a powerful person. A convicted criminal pleading for mercy from the judge—this is a supplicant engaged in supplication. When we come to God in supplication, we are recognizing his authority and his ability. He can because he is in charge and he can because he is equipped to do so.

Again there is good news here. Jesus told his listeners in Matthew 7, "If you who are evil know how to give good gifts to your children, how much more will your Father who is in heaven give good things to those who ask him!"

So our prayers start here: We talk to God about many matters but with full permission, even encouragement, to ask. If the gospel helps us recognize our utter dependence on God's mercy, asking God for the things we need is our way of recognizing his grace.

But we know this to be true as well: we should be asking others to pray for us. This becomes obvious when we make our way through the book of Acts and the letters of the apostles.

Let's consider three ways people might pray for you. I've chosen these examples because of the way they fit our full context of asking for help. First, 2 Corinthians 13:5-7:

> Examine yourselves, to see whether you are in the faith. Test yourselves. Or do you not realize this about yourselves, that Jesus Christ is in you?—unless indeed you fail to meet the test! I hope you will find out that we have not failed the test. But we pray to God that you may not do wrong—not that we may appear to have met the test, but that you may do what is right, though we may seem to have failed.

Here you are asking a friend to pray that you adhere to the gospel, that you are faith-filled and faithful from beginning to end. Eternal reward awaits those who persevere in the faith. Ask others to pray for this perseverance to be demonstrated in you.

Second, Colossians 4:2-4:

Continue steadfastly in prayer, being watchful in it with thanksgiving. At the same time, pray also for us, that God may open to us a door for the word, to declare the mystery of Christ, on account of which I am in prison—that I may make it clear, which is how I ought to speak.

Here we find Paul asking for prayer for practical things: that he be granted an open door for his ministry of evangelism. We pray similar things. You might in your current prayer life be asking God to give you a chance to speak of Jesus to an unbelieving friend or family member. This may be about an opportune time or a few minutes alone together without interruption or a conversational cue. Very simple, very practical. Paul could have asked that the church pray for his release from prison. That would have been a big prayer and a powerful answer. But instead, he asked them to pray for him to be able to conduct his ministry right where he was. Ask others to pray with you for seemingly ordinary things. We pray to the God who is known to turn ordinary beginnings into extraordinary outcomes.

Third, James 5:14-16:

Is anyone among you sick? Let him call for the elders of the church, and let them pray over him, anointing him with oil in the name of the Lord. And the prayer of faith will save the one who is sick, and the Lord will raise him up. And if he has committed sins, he will be forgiven. Therefore, confess your sins to one another and pray for one another, that you may be healed. The prayer of a righteous person has great power as it is working.

Here we are asking others, including the church's leaders, to pray for powerful things to happen in our body and in our spirit. Remember the context of James' writing. He lived in a time without germ theory, anesthesia, vaccines, or antibiotics. Doctors were essentially wound-bandagers and poultice-appliers and bone-setters; everything beyond that was a miracle. To be healed of illness and to be forgiven of sins—these were absolutely works of God. They still are. Miracles come in many forms. I would even suggest that we miss seeing vast numbers of these, having relegated them to categories like "common" or "explicable." Because we can now type genes, does this make their existence, their makeup, or their purpose, any less stunning? I grew up appreciating a song written and performed by Noel Paul Stuckey, in which he sang these words: "A scientist may tell you how the night turns into day/ but he can never take the wonder away." Ask others to pray with you for powerful things and together keep your eyes open for how those prayers are answered; you'll love that you can share the rejoicing!

When you can ask your friend to pray for your spiritual commitment, your practical needs, and powerful answers to big concerns, you are asking your friend to intercede—that is, to go between you and God. Let me affirm how important this is. Even the most disciplined follower of Christ will go through seasons of infirmity or discouragement; their prayers, when they can lift them at all, will be short and thin. This is where we can serve one another, stepping into the gap, adding to the weak brother's prayer with prayers of understanding and fellowship. This should be as apparent in the spiritual sense as it is in the physical. Humble, honest friends have said to me, "I can't get past this sin. I feel so powerless. What can I do?" Well, the first thing you can do when you have no strength of your own is to confess your weakness, and the second thing you can do is ask your brothers and sisters to pray with you that you may be renewed and your spiritual strength redoubled.

Ask a friend for practical help

The third thing you need to do is ask a friend for practical help.

This should be the easiest thing in the world, except that we are the proudest people in the world. From what I have read, people living on the street are better at asking for practical help than we are. We Christians, of all people, think it very important to present ourselves as having our acts together. This can descend into things like "cleanliness is next to godliness" or the Protestant work ethic—which if they aren't forms of legalism are certainly feeders of pride.

Asking others for practical help is both an admission that we cannot do it all and a way of letting others perform the ministry they are given to do. I'll speak more of spiritual gifts in a minute, but for now suffice it to say that if we elevate the gifts of teaching and preaching, say, above the gifts of mercy and helps, we don't really understand the body dynamic. If we insist on elevating the public gifts like teaching and do not give all in the body of Christ the chance to exercise their gifts, we are unbalanced at best and unhealthy at worst.

I previously noted that at the end of his second letter to Timothy, Paul asked his protégé to assist with some simple practical things: come quickly, bring my stuff. Paul was not above asking, and Timothy, though a pastor and teacher, was not above helping.

Let that be my charge here to you: Do not be above asking for even small help. And if you are asked to help, do not be above providing the help that is needed.

Ask a friend for powerful help

Finally, I want to consider something that may be a little outside the way you normally think of the help that your brothers and sisters can provide and encourage you to ask a friend for powerful help.

When we were considering prayer, we looked at the James 5 passage, where we read that "the prayer of a righteous person has great power as it is working." In the broad Christian context, power is something the Pentecostal or charismatic churches talk about freely, but the rest of us are, frankly, a bit spooked by the word. Yet the idea of power is all over the New Testament—through Jesus, of course, but also through the apostles and others. In fact, the core of what we have been talking about, which is the gospel, was explained by Paul to the Thessalonians this way:

> For we know, brothers loved by God, that he has chosen you, because our gospel came to you not only in word, but also in power and in the Holy Spirit and with full conviction.

The gospel is not only words and ideas. There is power behind it. And there is the Holy Spirit. And that is where the conversation shifts, isn't it? We're tentative about power, but we know we can't be tentative about the Holy Spirit. So as long as we're talking about the Holy Spirit's power, we're okay with it. But here's the thing: we cannot say that without adhering to the full counsel of Scripture, which tells us that the Holy Spirit dwells in us and that the Holy Spirit equips us each with spiritual gifts meant to serve and edify the fellowship of believers we call the body.

So here is where we can safely go when we ask a friend for powerful help: we can ask them to draw on the gifting they have been given by the power of the Holy Spirit and to use that gift to assist us in ways we cannot assist ourselves. From the gifts passages in Romans 12 and 1 Corinthians 12, we know that some have great faith, some encourage, some give generously, some lead, some show mercy, some administer, some teach. To be complete, there are other gifts listed there (prophecy, healing, miracles, tongues), but the definition and practice of these is discussed and sometimes disputed among churches today. That doesn't matter. The first part of the list is full enough. If doubts are raining down on you, go to someone with great faith and ask for powerful help in believing. If discouragement and even despair are knocking you down, go to someone who is gifted as an encourager and ask for words of promise and truth given by God for your uplifting. If circumstances have crushed you of late and left you without the resources you need, ask for help from one you know to be generous—for they will, by the power of the Holy Spirit, give as cheerful givers do. Are you seeing how this powerful help works? Ask for it.

the now and the not yet

THE KIND AND TYPICAL QUESTION we ask a friend when first meeting up with them hasn't changed in my lifetime. "How are you?" is so universally expressed that we don't expect a real answer. And so, "Fine" is what we get.

I see no reason to lament the superficial nature of this exchange in our culture. We all mean well enough. But I have come to recognize that the truest answer for any of us would sound like this: "I have no idea."

You may feel just fine today and discover tomorrow that the flu had been waiting to pounce on you; it just needed the night to set in. Or you may, like some noted athletes through the ages, be as fit as anyone could imagine, only to have your heart give out in a moment. For me, the truth despite my feeling fine was that a tumor was growing inside me. So slow was its development that the normal structures of my body accommodated its bullying presence, moving out of the way millimeter by millimeter. Like the erosion of a sinkhole, illness' effects are often not seen until catastrophe strikes.

Am I "fine"? Maybe. But like I said, I have no idea.

But there is another fact I know to be true. My health is not my greatest asset.

I balance the meats and sweets I eat with greens and nuts and berries. When I play golf, I walk as often as I possibly can. I'll work a day in the yard and enjoy "the good kind of tired" that comes of it. In these ways, I am healthy. But no one lives forever. One day this healthy body won't be able to fend off the weakness or disease that overtakes it. In my case, the large doses of radiation I received to fight this one cancer may feed the formation of another. I simply don't know.

When Bible teachers explain the kingdom of God as Jesus spoke of it, they describe it as "the now and the not yet." That is, the kingdom is among us even as we live here on earth, but its greatest fruition is in the future, when earth is restored and the road between here and heaven is wide open in both directions. Jesus will reign then, and there will be no more suffering, no more pain. I like the sound of that. More than that, I believe it!

My life is the same. I want to be increasingly present here and now. And God has permitted me to be. My tumor is gone—at least as far as the scans now tell us. I can do that work in the yard, play those rounds of golf, and spend wonderful hours with my wife, my children, my church, and my friends. But above and beyond all this, I can count on the salvation of Christ to carry me into eternity. Already I've written of how he is our ultimate provision, the man above all men, the lover of my soul. He is not providing only for my eternal future, though. I will find him in the bridge of time between now and then. He sends those I need, for the everyday help we all need, but he will send them also for the big help I'll likely need again someday. They'll come with specialized care, as doctors and nurses and techs. They'll come with only time to spend, as family and friends and Spirit-gifted ministers. In the physical end, they'll come and carry my body away, though that kind care will be God's provision for my loved ones more than for me. By then, I'll be with him.

Not so many days before writing these closing words, I stood with an old friend of the family. He is a man whose life has been blessed in all the ways men measure blessing. In these recent years, though, he has fought again and again the cancers that would kill him. Those cancers are winning, albeit slowly. He knows it. His body is frail, his white hair is thin. The bearing we all knew him for is gone. But his spiritual cornea is as strong as ever. His eyes are focused on Jesus. He speaks to me now not as a younger man, but as one who shares the knowledge that we are dust—two men grateful to be alive.

That day when we stood together, he looked at me intently and reminded me of what I should very much know by now: "We keep hanging in there. But if we don't, it doesn't matter. We're going home. We're going home." In his voice—still the voice I've always known—was the provision of God again. Through him, the Lord had given me the words I need to hear, as often as possible, from now until the not yet.

still counting

PERHAPS MY GREATEST DISAPPOINTMENT in writing this book is that I do not have a comprehensive list of every person who helped me through my year of cancer. I am sure you have gathered that it was far, far more than a hundred.

What I can do here at least is thank those who helped me in reading through the manuscript and preparing the book for you to read. Those include several people already mentioned in these pages: my wife Laura, my sister Kendra, and Barbara Jacobus. Laura was my fact checker, while Kendra and Barbara helped catch errors big and small. Another friend in this endeavor was my Links Players colleague Lewis Greer, who shares both my love of the game and my love of writing. He always helps me keep a watchful eye toward clean copy.

But what I have learned is that counting on people is far more significant than just counting them. I am blessed that these friends are among the so many I can count on.